Complete
Understanding and
TREATMENT OF CHOLERA

Louis J. Cole

Table of Contents

CHAPTER ONE 3
  Understanding Cholera 3
  The signs and symptoms of cholera 3
  Spread of Cholera 7
  Risk Factors and Cholera Complications 9

CHAPTER TWO 12
  Possible Cholera Complications 12

CHAPTER THREE 16
  Treatment of Cholera 16
  Intravenous Fluids (IV) 18
  Preventive Actions 21

CHAPTER FOUR 23
  Medication for Cholera 23
  Supportive Care for Cholera Patients 30
  Relaxation and Observation 33

CHAPTER FIVE 37
Preventing Cholera 37
Safe Water and Sanitation Practices 45

CHAPTER SIX 53
Coping with Cholera: Extended Consequences and Handling ... 53
Management and Recovery 56

CHAPTER SEVEN 62
Cholera Outbreaks and Public Health Measures 62

THE END 70

CHAPTER ONE
Understanding Cholera
What is the cholera virus?

Acute diarrheal sickness known as cholera is brought on by an intestinal Vibrio cholerae infection. Although the infection is usually mild or symptomless, it can occasionally be serious and potentially fatal. If severe cases are not treated right once, they can quickly cause shock and dehydration.

The signs and symptoms of cholera

After infection, cholera symptoms might develop anywhere from a few hours to five days later.

Typical signs and symptoms include of:

Severe Diarrhea: Frequently referred to as "rice-water stools" because of their pale, milky consistency.

vomiting: This has the potential to cause more dehydration.

Elevated Heart Rate: Owing to dehydration.

Loss of Skin Elasticity: When skin is pinched, it keeps its tent shape.

Dry Mucous Membranes: nose, throat, and mouth are dry.

Fluid loss is the cause of low blood pressure.

Thirst: A strong desire to consume liquids.

Muscle cramps: Caused by an imbalance in electrolytes.

Dehydration can cause restlessness or irritability, especially in young children.

If left untreated in extreme cases, cholera can cause:

Severe Dehydration and Shock: These conditions have an hourly death rate.

The bacteria Vibrio cholerae is the cause of cholera.

Vibrio cholerae is the bacteria that causes cholera. Diarrhea is caused by the cholera toxin that the bacteria generate, which causes the intestinal lining cells to discharge more water. The following are the primary causes of cholera:

Drinking water tainted with the bacteria is the main source of the problem.

Consuming tainted food, especially seafood, is known as contaminated food.

Poor Sanitation: The bacterium can spread more easily when there is insufficient water treatment, poor sanitation, and inadequate hygiene habits.

Spread of Cholera

The usual means of transmission for cholera are:

Consuming Toxicity-Infected Water: Sipping water tainted by excrement harboring the Vibrio cholerae bacteria.

Eating Contaminated Food: Eating food that has come into contact with tainted water or has been handled by sick people.

Person-to-Person Contact: Direct contact with an infected person's feces can transmit cholera, however this is less likely.

Among the preventive actions are:

Boiling or treating water before drinking is one way to ensure that it is safe to consume.

Using soap to wash your hands is part of practicing proper sanitation and hygiene, especially after using the restroom and before handling food.

Keeping meals well cooked and steering clear of raw or undercooked seafood are safe food practices.

Immunization: In regions where cholera is endemic or during outbreaks, cholera vaccinations are advised and readily available.

Comprehending these facets of cholera can facilitate the efficient prevention and management of epidemics.

Risk Factors and Cholera Complications

Who Is Most Likely to Contract Cholera?

The following variables raise the chance of catching cholera:

Living in Unsanitary Areas: Communities that suffer from inadequate water treatment, unsanitary conditions, and dense population density are more vulnerable.

Exposure to Contaminated Water Sources: Those who bathe and drink from untreated water sources, like rivers or lakes, are particularly vulnerable.

Traveling to Cholera-Endemic Areas: There is an increased danger for visitors going to cholera-endemic or outbreak-affected areas.

Eating food that has been contaminated with cholera bacteria increases the chance of contracting the disease. Seafood is particularly susceptible to this problem.

Underlying Health Conditions: People who are malnourished, have compromised immune systems, or suffer from long-term illnesses are particularly vulnerable.

Lack of Access to Healthcare: The risk and severity of cholera might be increased by a lack of timely and sufficient medical treatment.

Children and the Elderly: Due to their immature or compromised immune systems, young children and the elderly may be particularly vulnerable.

CHAPTER TWO
Possible Cholera Complications

Serious consequences from cholera can arise if treatment is not received, such as:

Severe Dehydration: Severe dehydration can be fatal if there is a sudden loss of fluids and electrolytes.

Severe thirst, dry skin, sunken eyes, decreased urine production, and lethargic behavior are symptoms of severe dehydration.

Electrolyte imbalance: When vital electrolytes like potassium, sodium, and chloride are lost, it can lead to:

Painful contractions of the muscles known as cramps.

Shock: Low blood pressure and insufficient blood supply to the organs, which may cause organ failure.

Cardiac arrhythmia: Loss of potassium causing irregular heartbeats.

Renal Failure: When the kidneys are unable to filter waste materials from the blood, severe dehydration can cause acute kidney damage and renal failure.

Hypoglycemia: Dangerously low blood sugar levels can result from severe dehydration and malnutrition, particularly in young patients.

Death: Severe cholera can be lethal, sometimes within hours, if treatment is delayed and ineffective.

Rapid rehydration therapy, medicines in severe cases, and preventive measures including bettering water quality, sanitation, and hygiene standards are all important components of effective cholera management.

CHAPTER THREE
Treatment of Cholera

The Cornerstone of Cholera Treatment: Rehydration Therapy

Rehydration therapy is the first and most important line of treatment for cholera. Replacing lost fluids and electrolytes is the aim in order to avoid shock and dehydration.

Solution for Oral Rehydration (ORS)

Easy to give, Oral Rehydration Solution (ORS) is a low-cost, straightforward treatment:

Composition: ORS usually consists of a specific blend of sugars and salts that, when dissolved in purified water, improve the body's ability to absorb fluids.

Administration: ORS is usually administered in tiny doses, particularly following each loose bowel movement. ORS is frequently enough to replenish fluids in mild to moderate episodes of dehydration.

Effectiveness: By quickly replenishing patients' electrolyte balance and rehydrating them, ORS can save around 90% of cholera-related deaths.

Availability: ORS packets can be manufactured at home or given at medical facilities, and they are generally accessible. Six level teaspoons of sugar and half a level teaspoon of salt dissolved in one liter of clean water can be used to make a DIY treatment in an emergency.

Intravenous Fluids (IV)

Intravenous (IV) fluids are required in severe cases of cholera when the dehydration is too severe for ORS alone:

Use: IV fluids are administered to patients who are too dehydrated to ingest fluids on their own, are in shock, or require immediate fluid replacement.

Types of IV Fluids: Normal saline or other balanced electrolyte solutions can be used in place of Ringer's lactate solution, which is the preferred option.

Administration: In order to facilitate quicker rehydration, medical personnel inject IV fluids directly into the bloodstream. The patient's weight, age, and degree of dehydration are taken into consideration while determining the appropriate volume and pace of fluid delivery.

Monitoring: In order to modify the fluid rate and keep an eye out for any potential consequences, such fluid overload, patients receiving IV fluids need to be continuously monitored.

Extra Measures of Treatment

Although rehydration therapy is the mainstay, additional therapies could be used:

Antibiotics: Antibiotics can lessen the length and intensity of an illness in cases ranging from moderate to severe. Antibiotics like ciprofloxacin, azithromycin, and doxycycline are frequently utilized. To lower the bacterial burden and stop spread, antibiotics are especially crucial in severe cases and outbreaks.

Zinc Supplements: Zinc supplements help youngsters recover more quickly from diarrhea and shorten its length.

Nutritional Support: It's critical to maintain nutrition, particularly for young people and those who are malnourished. Recuperation is aided by continuous feeding with readily digested meals.

Preventive Actions

In order to supplement therapy and stop further outbreaks:

Providing a source of clean drinking water is known as "access to clean water."

Sanitation and Hygiene: enhancing the infrastructure for proper sanitation and encouraging the use of soap and water for handwashing.

Immunization: In endemic areas or during outbreaks, cholera vaccinations are advised and readily available.

Prompt and proper rehydration therapy, supportive care, and preventive actions to lower the risk of future infections are necessary for effective cholera treatment.

CHAPTER FOUR
Medication for Cholera
antibiotics

When treating cholera, antibiotics can be a valuable addition to rehydration therapy, especially in more severe cases. By reducing the length and intensity of symptoms as well as the time that bacteria are released in the feces, they aid in slowing the disease's spread.

Commonly Used Antibiotics:

Doxycycline:

Dosage: 300 mg as a single dose for adults, or 2-4 mg/kg for kids, according on weight and age.

Benefits: Generally well-tolerated and effective against Vibrio cholerae.

Zithromycin:

Dosage: Adults should take one gram, while children should take 20 mg/kg.

Benefits: Reduces symptoms and bacterial shedding; safe for youngsters and pregnant women.

Ciprofloxacine:

Dosage: Adults: 500 mg twice day for three days, or 1 gram in one dosage; children: 20 mg/kg in one dose.

Benefits: Generally accessible and efficient, however resistance may be a problem in some areas.

Tetracycline:

Adults should take 500 mg four times a day for three days.

Benefits: Good, however owing to possible adverse effects, not advised for pregnant women or children under the age of eight.

Taking Antibiotic Use Into Account:

Indications: Saved for extreme situations, susceptible groups (children, expectant mothers), and during epidemics to stop the spread of the disease.

Resistance: To guarantee the efficacy of selected antibiotics, it is essential to monitor local trends of resistance.

Additional Drugs

Anti-diarrhea

General Information: It is not advised to treat cholera with antidiarrheal drugs like loperamide. By postponing the pathogen's excretion, these drugs have the potential to exacerbate the illness by slowing down the removal of microorganisms from the intestines.

Supplements containing zinc:

Use: Suggested for kids suffering from cholera to lessen the length and intensity of diarrhea.

Dosage: 10 mg per day for children under 6 months old, and 20 mg per day for children aged 6 to 14 months.

Benefits: Zinc supports quicker healing by enhancing immunological response and intestinal barrier function.

Extra Helpful Actions:

Nutritional Support: To maintain nutrition and aid in recuperation, it's critical to keep nursing and to provide children age-appropriate meals.

Probiotics: Although not a recommended course of therapy, probiotics may assist in reestablishing a healthy balance of gut flora after cholera and its treatment have disrupted it.

In brief

The mainstay of effective cholera treatment is early oral and intravenous rehydration therapy, which may be augmented with the proper use of antibiotics in more severe patients. Children can benefit from zinc supplementation, but antidiarrheal drugs should be avoided. Recuperation can be accelerated by supportive interventions like sustained feeding and potentially probiotics. Prevention is still the key to managing and averting cholera epidemics. This includes having access to clean water, sanitary conditions, and immunizations.

Supportive Care for Cholera Patients

dietary assistance

One of the most important aspects of cholera patients' supportive care is proper diet. Sustaining a healthy diet boosts the immune system and expedites healing.

Sustaining Food:

Children: It's critical to keep breastfeeding newborns. Antibodies and vital nutrients from breast milk help bolster an infant's immune system. Age-appropriate diets should be continued for older kids.

Adults: Patients should keep eating everything they are able to. Foods ought to be nutrient-dense and easily digested.

Food Types:

The first line of nutritional treatment is oral rehydration solution (ORS), which aids in electrolyte replacement and hydration.

Foods That Are Easily Digested: These include bread, rice, potatoes, bananas, and oatmeal.

Foods High in Protein: As soon as the patient feels hungry again, you can start adding in eggs, yogurt, and lean meats.

Fruits and vegetables: Offer vital minerals and vitamins. To reduce the possibility of contamination, these should be cooked thoroughly.

Steer clear of specific foods:

Dairy Products: With the exception of yogurt, patients suffering from transient lactose intolerance may experience worsening diarrhea from dairy products.

Foods that are high in fat and spice should be avoided because they can irritate the intestines and stomach.

Relaxation and Observation

Cholera patients need to be closely monitored and given enough rest to fully recover.

Relax:

Relevance: Sleep preserves energy needed for healing and aids in the body's healing process.

Setting: A serene, well-kept setting is ideal for patients. Comfortable bedding and a quiet room are two things that can help you sleep better.

Observing:

Hydration Status: It's critical to keep an ongoing eye on the patient's level of hydration. Look out for symptoms of dehydration, such as decreased urine output, sunken eyes, dry mouth, and turgor in the skin.

Vital Signs: Keep a regular eye on your vital signs, including your blood pressure, heart rate, and breathing rate. This aids in the early detection of any indicators of shock or severe dehydration.

Electrolyte Levels: If at all feasible, monitor electrolyte levels—particularly those of sodium, potassium, and chloride—through blood testing. This aids in preventing problems like hypokalemia or hyponatremia.

Fluid Intake and outflow: Record the amount of fluid intake and outflow to ensure the patient is rehydrating adequately. This includes measuring urine production and the number of feces.

General Condition: Look out for any changes in the patient's general condition, including alertness, responsiveness, and overall physical well-being. This assists in assessing the success of treatment and making appropriate modifications.

In brief

Supportive therapy for cholera patients entails both dietary support and watchful monitoring. Adequate nutrition helps patients restore strength and recover faster, while careful monitoring of hydration status, vital signs, and general condition ensures timely intervention and adjustment of treatments. Rest is equally vital as it allows the body to recuperate. Together, these supportive care strategies are critical for the successful recovery of cholera patients.

CHAPTER FIVE
Preventing Cholera

Immunization (The Best Way to Prevent Cholera)

Immunization is one of the best ways to avoid cholera, particularly in high-risk areas and during epidemics. Immunostimulating the body against the Vibrio cholerae bacteria lowers the risk of serious illness caused by cholera vaccinations.

Different Cholera Vaccine Types

Cholera vaccines come in two primary varieties:

OCVs, or oral cholera vaccines, were killed:

Dukoral:

The cholera toxin component and dead Vibrio cholerae O1 bacteria are present in this vaccine.

Dosage: Given 1-6 weeks apart in two doses for adults and children over the age of six, and in three doses for children ages two to six.

Effectiveness: Offers defense for approximately a week following the second dosage and continues for roughly two years.

Special Notes: In addition to preventing traveler's diarrhea, dukoral also guards against enterotoxigenic Escherichia coli (ETEC).

Euvichol and Shanchol:

The O1 and O139 serogroups of dead Vibrio cholerae are present in these vaccinations.

Dosage: Given in two doses spaced two to six weeks apart.

Effectiveness: Up to three years of protection are possible, beginning around a week after the second dosage.

Accessibility: Because these vaccinations are less expensive, they are utilized more frequently in large-scale immunization campaigns.

Vaccine against live attenuated oral cholera:

Vaxchora:

Description: Vibrio cholerae O1 live, weakened strain is included in this vaccination.

Dosage: One oral dosage administered.

Effectiveness: After immunization, protection starts to take effect within ten days and lasts for at least three months.

Special Notes: Especially available in the US, this medication is authorized for use by anyone between the ages of 2 and 64 who are visiting cholera-affected areas.

Recommended Vaccinations

Areas at High Risk:

It is advised that those who reside in or plan to visit regions where cholera is endemic or experiencing an outbreak get vaccinated. This covers a portion of Haiti, South Asia, and Africa.

In the Event of an Outbreak:

During cholera outbreaks, mass vaccination efforts can be used to contain and stop the disease's spread. Governments and health groups frequently organize these programs.

Particular Populations:

Travelers: Those who plan to visit areas impacted by cholera should think about being vaccinated, especially if they won't have easy access to sanitary facilities and clean water.

Healthcare and Aid Workers: It may be recommended that those who work in cholera-prone areas or assist with outbreak response get vaccinated.

Populations in refugee camps and conflict zones are more vulnerable because of the overcrowding and poor access to sanitary facilities and clean water.

Regular Immunization in endemic regions:

Routine immunization may be a part of public health initiatives to lower the incidence of cholera in places where outbreaks occur frequently.

In brief

Immunization has a vital role in cholera prevention, especially in high-risk areas and during epidemics. There are several cholera vaccine varieties, each with distinct dosages and effectiveness profiles, such as dead oral vaccinations and a live attenuated oral vaccine. The main targets of vaccination recommendations include communities in endemic areas, visitors, healthcare workers, and high-risk groups. In addition to other preventive measures including better sanitation, water, and hygiene practices, immunization against cholera is essential for lowering the disease's worldwide burden.

Safe Water and Sanitation Practices

Sources of Clean Water Are Important

The prevention of cholera and other waterborne illnesses depends on having access to clean, safe water. The bacterium that causes cholera, Vibrio cholerae, primarily spreads through contaminated water. Reducing the likelihood of cholera outbreaks can be achieved by ensuring that water sources are safe and uncontaminated.

Potable Water That Is Safe:

Methods of Treatment: In order to eradicate or destroy microorganisms, water must be treated. Boiling, chlorinating, filtering, and sun disinfection (SODIS) are typical techniques.

Use piped water systems, wells, or boreholes as protected sources. Lakes and other open water sources ought to be avoided unless they have been treated.

Correct Storage:

Clean Containers: To avoid contamination, water should be kept in clean, covered containers.

Prevent Recontamination: Use containers with narrow necks and refrain from using your hands or other filthy things to touch the water or the container's inside.

Water Systems in Communities:

Frequent Maintenance: Make sure that municipal water systems are appropriately cared for and routinely inspected for pollution.

Raising Community Awareness: Inform the public about the value of using treated water and upholding hygienic water storage methods.

Suitable Hygiene Procedures

In order to stop the spread of cholera and other infectious diseases, good hygiene habits are crucial. These procedures aid in interrupting the infections' cycle of transmission.

Hand hygiene:

Importance: One of the best strategies to stop the spread of cholera is to regularly wash your hands with soap and clean water.

Important Times to Hand Wash:

prior to consuming or cooking food.

following a bathroom visit.

following the cleansing of a child who has urinated.

prior to giving a child food.

following contact with animals or animal feces.

Facilities for Sanitation:

Access to restrooms: Make use of and maintain appropriate restrooms and latrines. Make sure these spaces are hygienic and operational.

Waste Management: In order to avoid contaminating water sources, dispose of human waste appropriately. Using latrines and making sure sewage systems are operational and maintained are part of this.

Keeping Food Clean:

Handwash before handling food to ensure safe handling practices. Food should be well cooked, especially seafood, and eaten hot.

Storage: To keep flies and other pests away from food, keep it covered.

Cleaning Fruits and Vegetables: Before eating, wash fruits and vegetables in safe, treated water.

Cleanliness of the Environment:

Waste Management: Make sure that rubbish is gathered and handled effectively. Properly dispose of household waste.

Cleaning Environments: Make sure your living spaces are contaminant-free and spotless. Keep surfaces that come into contact with food and water clean on a regular basis.

In brief

The prevention of cholera is largely dependent on having access to clean water as well as good sanitation and hygiene practices. The risk of cholera and other waterborne diseases can be decreased by ensuring safe drinking water through treated and protected sources, upholding good hygiene practices like frequent handwashing and safe food handling, and making use of appropriate sanitation facilities. Public education and community involvement are also essential for advancing these behaviors and stopping cholera epidemics.

CHAPTER SIX
Coping with Cholera: Extended Consequences and Handling

Although cholera is primarily an acute illness, those who are recovering must receive the right care and attention to guarantee a full recovery and avoid complications. Although there are rarely long-term consequences, the experience of extreme dehydration and its effects can have an impact on a person's health and wellbeing.

Effects of Cholera Over Time

Inadequate Dietary Resources:

Malnutrition: Prolonged diarrhea, particularly in children, can cause a substantial loss of nutrients. Nutritional supplementation may be necessary for recovering individuals to regain strength and normal growth patterns.

Deficiencies in vitamins and minerals: When diarrhea is severe, the body loses vitamins and electrolytes like potassium, salt, and chloride, which can lead to imbalances that need to be corrected.

Issues with Growth and Development:

Children: Repeated bouts of cholera or severe cases might damage a child's growth and cognitive development. Ensuring sufficient nutrition and health care post-recovery is vital.

Psychological Impact:

Stress and Anxiety: The experience of a severe sickness can be traumatic, especially in locations with frequent outbreaks. Supportive treatment, including mental health help, may be needed.

Chronic Health Issues:

Persistent Diarrhea: In some circumstances, especially in

malnourished or immunocompromised persons, diarrhea may remain for a prolonged duration, requiring constant medical attention.

Management and Recovery

Rehydration and Nutrition:

Ongoing Hydration: Continue to encourage fluid intake even after the acute phase to ensure complete rehydration.

Balanced Diet: To aid in the body's strength reconstruction, offer a diet high in vital nutrients. Make sure to eat lots of fruits, veggies, healthy grains, and lean proteins.

Supplementation: If there has been a significant loss of nutrients, doctors may advise taking supplements, particularly for young patients.

Medical Aftercare:

Frequent Check-Ups: Make follow-up appointments to track your progress and take care of any unresolved medical concerns.

Monitoring Development and Growth: It's critical to routinely keep an eye on a child's developmental milestones and growth indicators.

Support for Mental Health:

Counseling Services: Having access to mental health specialists can assist people in managing the psychological effects of their illness.

Community Support Groups: Attending a community support group can provide both practical recovery advice and emotional support.

Preventive actions:

Vaccination: To avoid additional outbreaks, people who live in or are visiting high-risk areas should think about getting vaccinated against cholera.

Emphasize the value of maintaining proper cleanliness habits in order to ward off reinfections. This covers using clean water, handling food safely, and washing your hands properly.

Enhancing Public Health:

Better Water and Sanitation Access: Promote and assist neighborhood initiatives to upgrade the infrastructure for water and sanitation.

Engage in or advocate for health education initiatives that disseminate information about cholera prevention and good hygiene habits.

In brief

Dealing with the short- and long-term health effects of cholera as well as its recovery requires managing both of these issues. A complete recovery depends on ensuring adequate fluids, nutritional assistance, follow-up treatment from the doctor, and psychological support. In areas where cholera is endemic, preventive measures—such as immunization and better hygiene practices—are essential for controlling the disease and averting further infections. Support from the community and the healthcare system is crucial for promoting recovery and strengthening defenses against cholera epidemics in the future.

CHAPTER SEVEN
Cholera Outbreaks and Public Health Measures

Comprehending Cholera Epidemics

When there is an abrupt rise in the number of cholera cases in a particular location, it is known as an outbreak. Conditions including poor sanitation, contaminated water supplies, and crowded living quarters are frequently linked to outbreaks of Vibrio cholerae.

Strategies in Public Health to Manage and Avoid Cholera Epidemics

A combination of long-term preventive measures and quick response actions is needed to effectively manage cholera epidemics.

Monitoring and Prompt Identification:

Monitoring Systems: To identify cases of cholera early, put in place reliable monitoring systems. This include routine reports from health facilities and monitoring of the quality of the water.

Create Rapid Response Teams: To look into and act quickly on suspected cases of cholera, establish rapid response teams.

Emergency Reaction:

Treatment Centers: Establish cholera treatment centers (CTCs) or units (CTUs) to offer afflicted parties prompt medical attention. Make sure patients have all the resources they need, including IV fluids, antibiotics, and ORS.

Community Health Workers: Educate the public, detect cases, and support efforts at prevention and treatment by training and placing community health workers.

Interventions related to water, sanitation, and hygiene (WASH):

Enable people to have access to clean drinking water. This could entail putting emergency water supply systems in place, chlorinating water sources, and giving out pills that purify water.

Sanitation Facilities: Build and maintain sewage systems and latrines to improve sanitation. Take care to dispose of rubbish in a safe manner to avoid contamination.

Hygiene Promotion: Through community education programs, encourage the use of soap when washing hands, safe food preparation, and appropriate disposal of garbage.

Campaigns for Vaccination:

Oral Cholera Vaccines (OCVs): To offer rapid protection against cholera, conduct widespread immunization programs in high-risk locations. It is possible to employ vaccines such as Dukoral, Euvichol, and Shanchol.

Targeted Vaccination: Concentrate on immunizing susceptible groups, such as those residing in urban slums, camps for refugees, and areas where epidemics are still occurring.

Participation in the Community and Education:

Public Awareness Campaigns: Spread knowledge about cholera prevention, symptoms, and the value of receiving treatment as soon as possible using a variety of media channels.

Community Involvement: To guarantee local buy-in and sustainability, involve community leaders and groups in the planning and execution of cholera control measures.

Partnerships and Coordination:

Multisectoral Approach: To coordinate efforts and resources, work with local communities, international health organizations, non-governmental organizations (NGOs), and government agencies.

Logistics and Supply Chain Management: Make certain that the impacted communities receive clean water, medical supplies, and sanitation supplies in an expedient manner.

Prolonged Preventive Actions:

Infrastructure Improvement: To ensure sustainable access to clean water and appropriate waste management, invest in long-term upgrades to the water and sanitation infrastructure.

Strengthening Health Systems: To enhance disease surveillance, the ability to respond to outbreaks, and the provision of healthcare overall, health systems should be strengthened.

Environmental Management: Use environmental management techniques, such as appropriate drainage systems to avoid water contamination and stagnation, to lower the risk of cholera.

THE END

www.ingramcontent.com/pod-product-compliance
Lightning Source LLC
Chambersburg PA
CBHW071842210526
45479CB00001B/249